UPDOG

DEADLY DISEASES

MALARIA

An Ongoing Threat

Brianna Kaiser

Lerner Publications ◆ Minneapolis

Lerner Publications Company
An imprint of Lerner Publishing Group, Inc.
241 First Avenue North
Minneapolis, MN 55401 USA

For reading levels and more information, look up this title at www.lernerbooks.com.

Main body text set in ITC Franklin Gothic Std.
Typeface provided by Adobe Systems.

Designer: Mary Ross
Lerner team: Sue Marquis

Library of Congress Cataloging-in-Publication Data

Names: Kaiser, Brianna, 1996– author.
Title: Malaria : an ongoing threat / Brianna Kaiser.
Description: Minneapolis, : Lerner Publications , [2022] | Series: Deadly diseases (UpDog Books) | Includes bibliographical references and index. | Audience: Ages 8–11 | Audience: Grades 2–3 | Summary: "Every year, mosquitoes pass parasites that cause malaria to hundreds of millions of people, and hundreds of thousands die. See how the disease works and the ways doctors and scientists fight malaria"— Provided by publisher.
Identifiers: LCCN 2020043818 (print) | LCCN 2020043819 (ebook) | ISBN 9781728428369 (library binding) | ISBN 9781728431253 (paperback) | ISBN 9781728430638 (ebook)
Subjects: LCSH: Malaria—Juvenile literature.
Classification: LCC RC157 .K35 2022 (print) | LCC RC157 (ebook) | DDC 616.9/362—dc23

LC record available at https://lccn.loc.gov/2020043818
LC ebook record available at https://lccn.loc.gov/2020043819

Manufactured in the United States of America
1-49373-49477-1/22/2021

Table of Contents

Malaria

A mosquito bites a person.

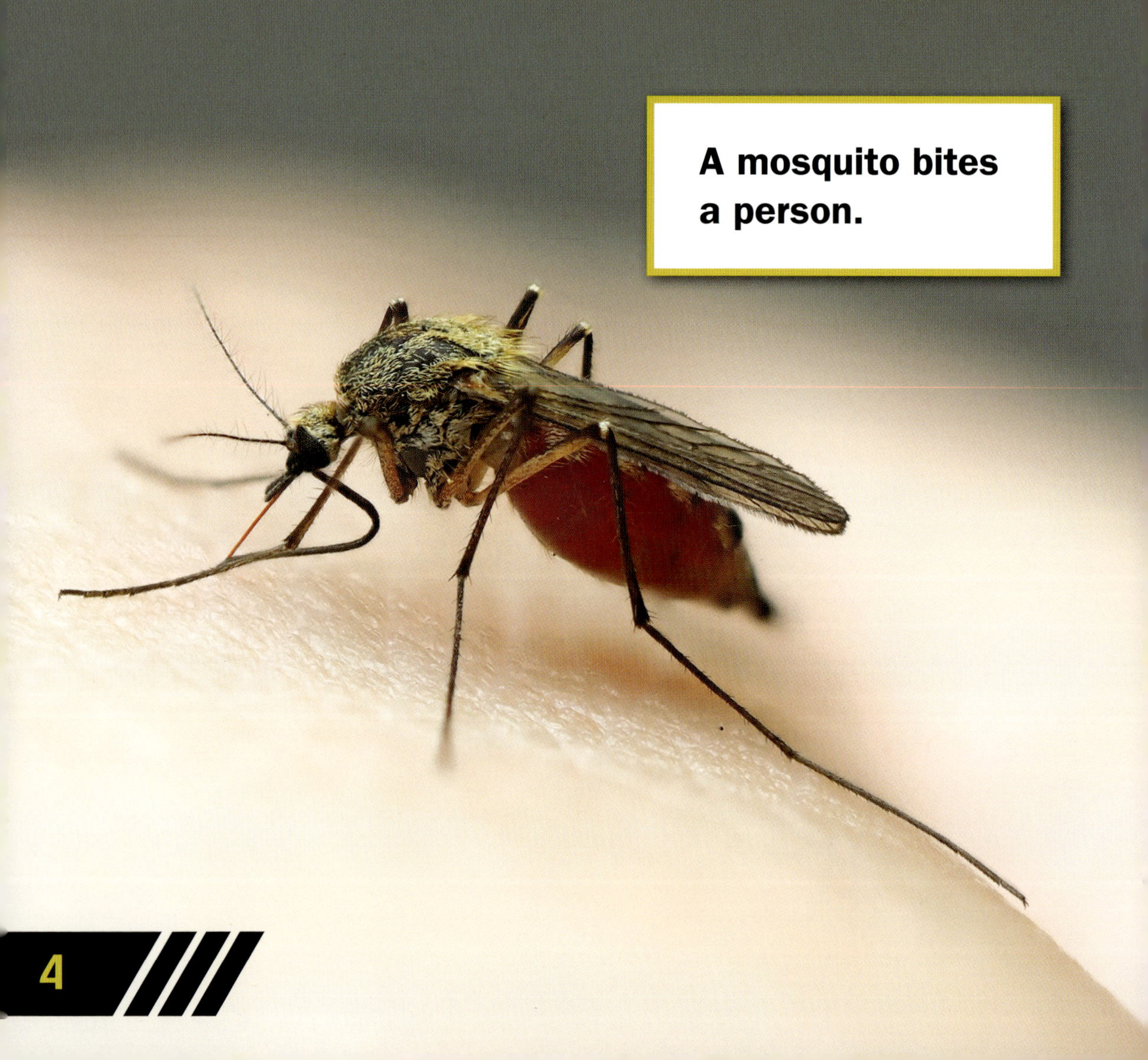

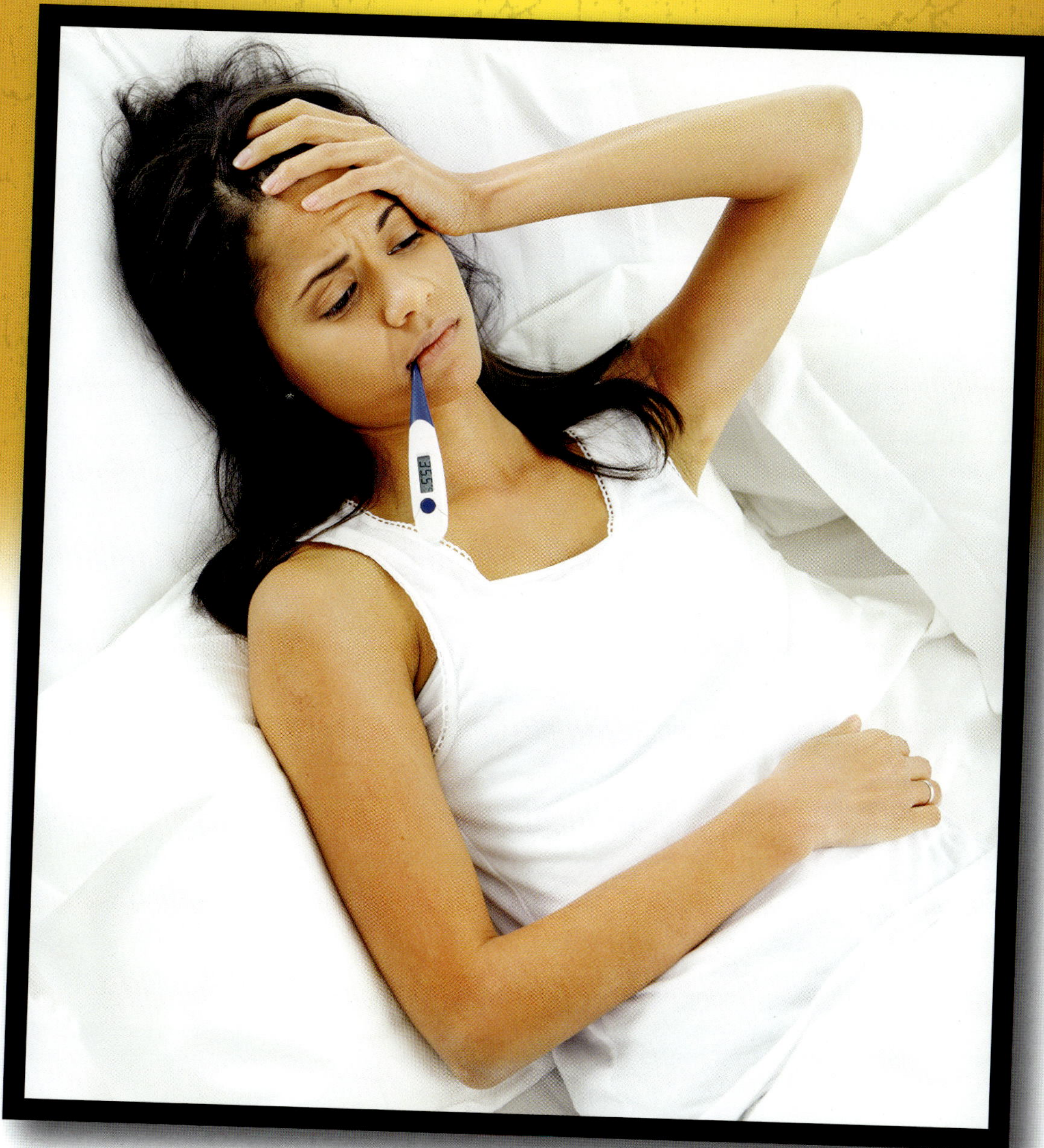

Two weeks later, the person feels sick.
Is it malaria?

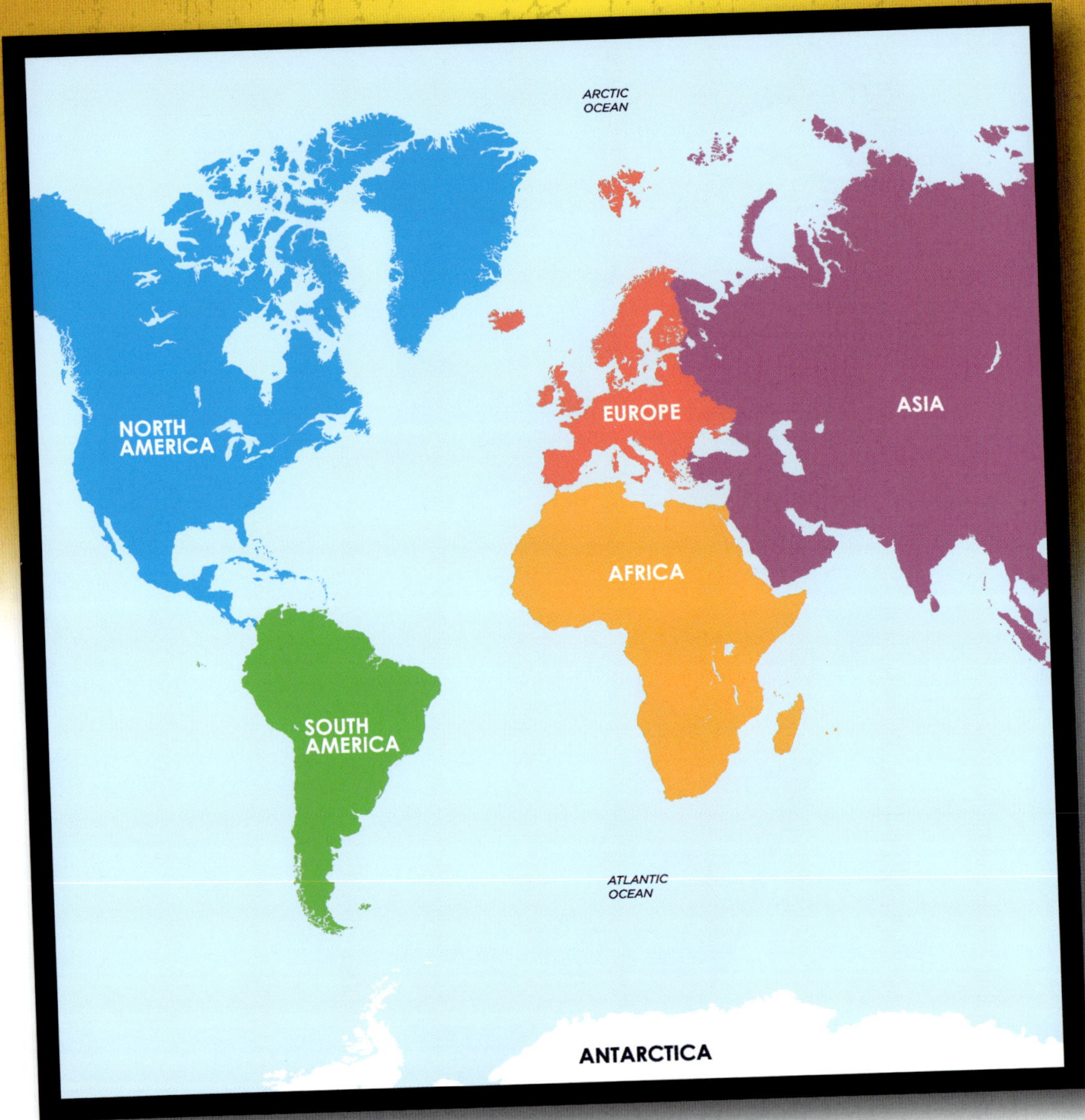

The disease is common in many warm places.

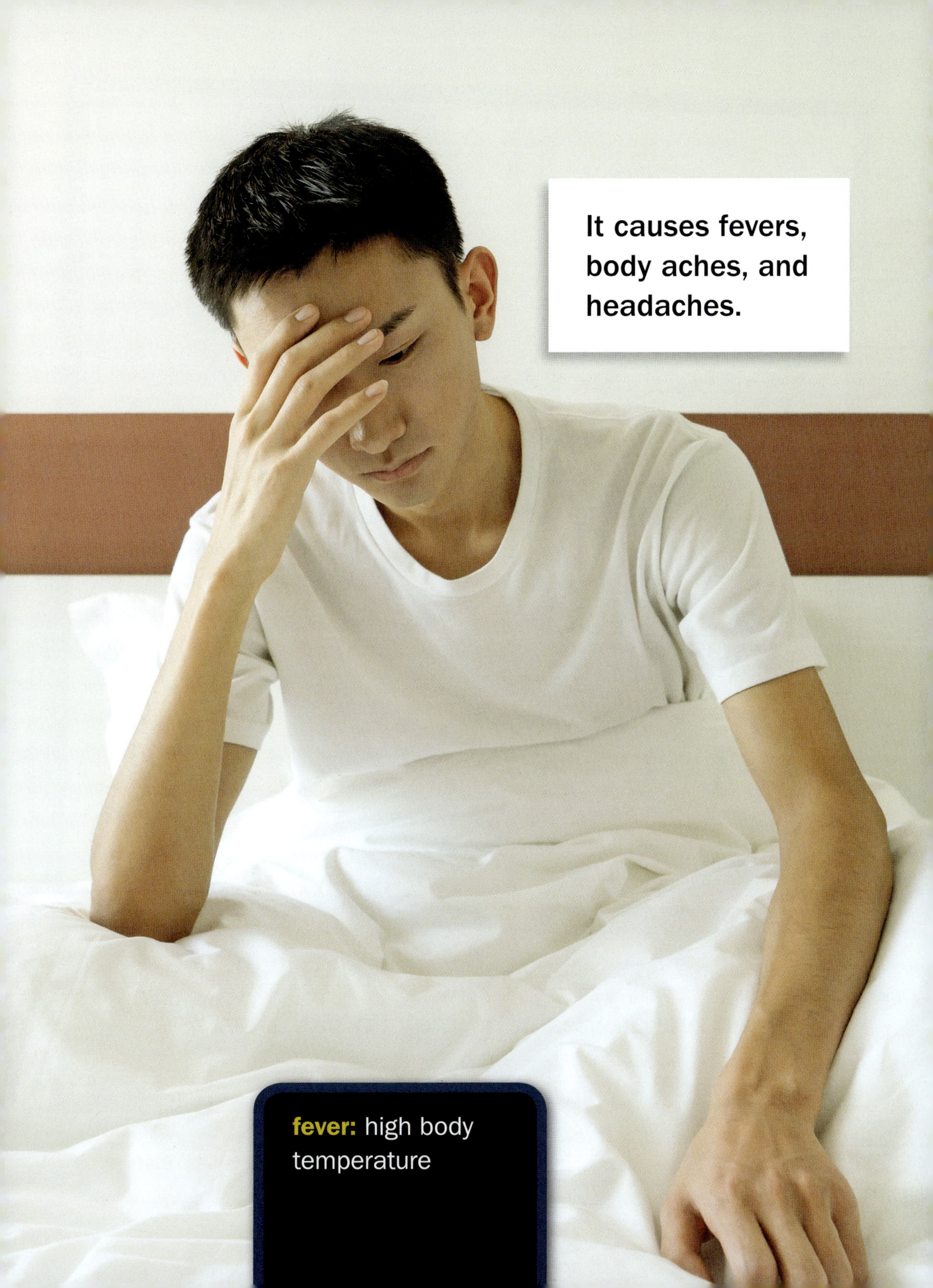

It causes fevers, body aches, and headaches.

fever: high body temperature

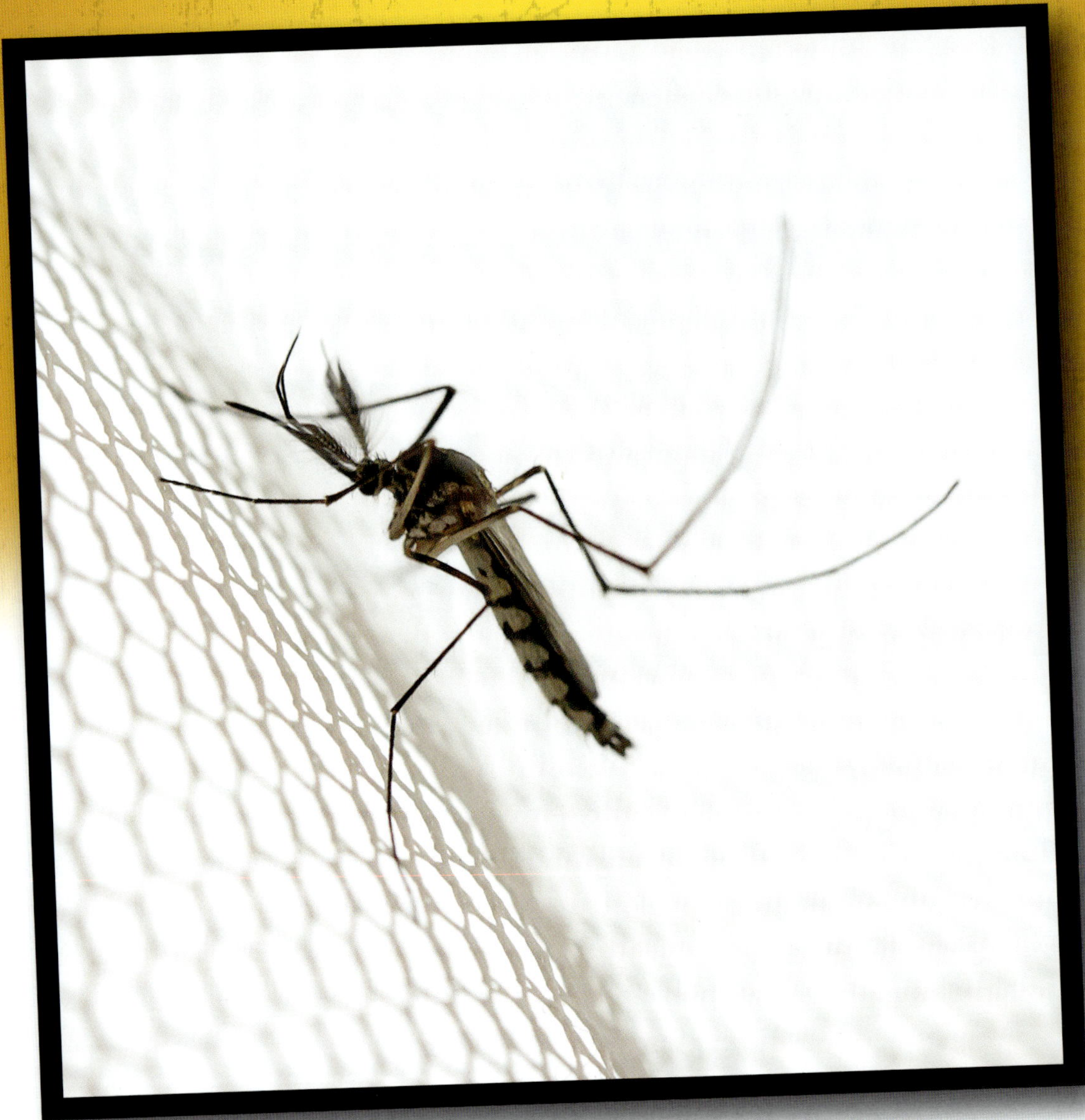

Some mosquitoes carry malaria parasites.

parasite: a living thing that lives on or in another living thing

The insects bite and pass on some of the parasites.

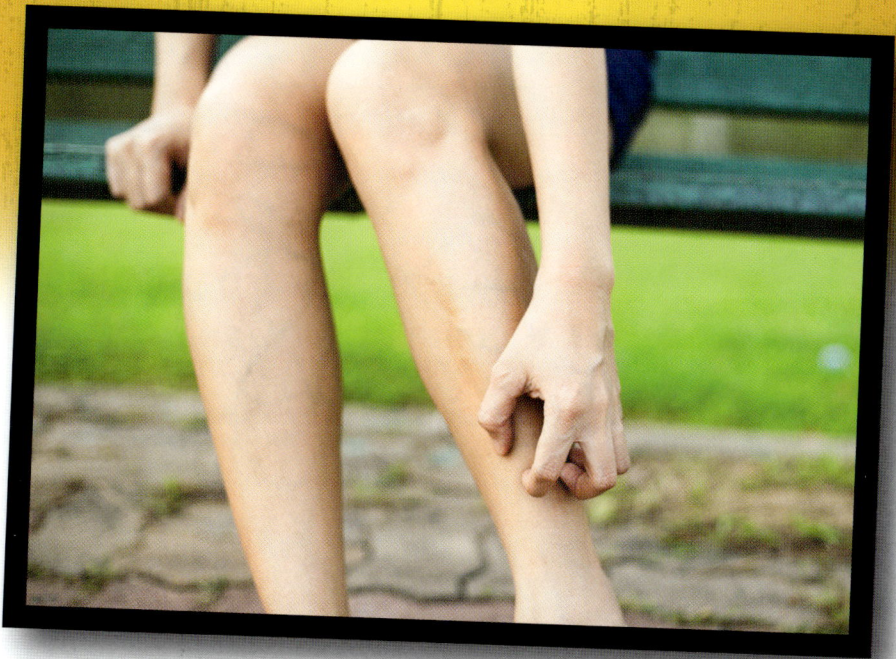

UP NEXT!

The Disease Spreads.

The History of Malaria

Malaria has affected people for thousands of years.

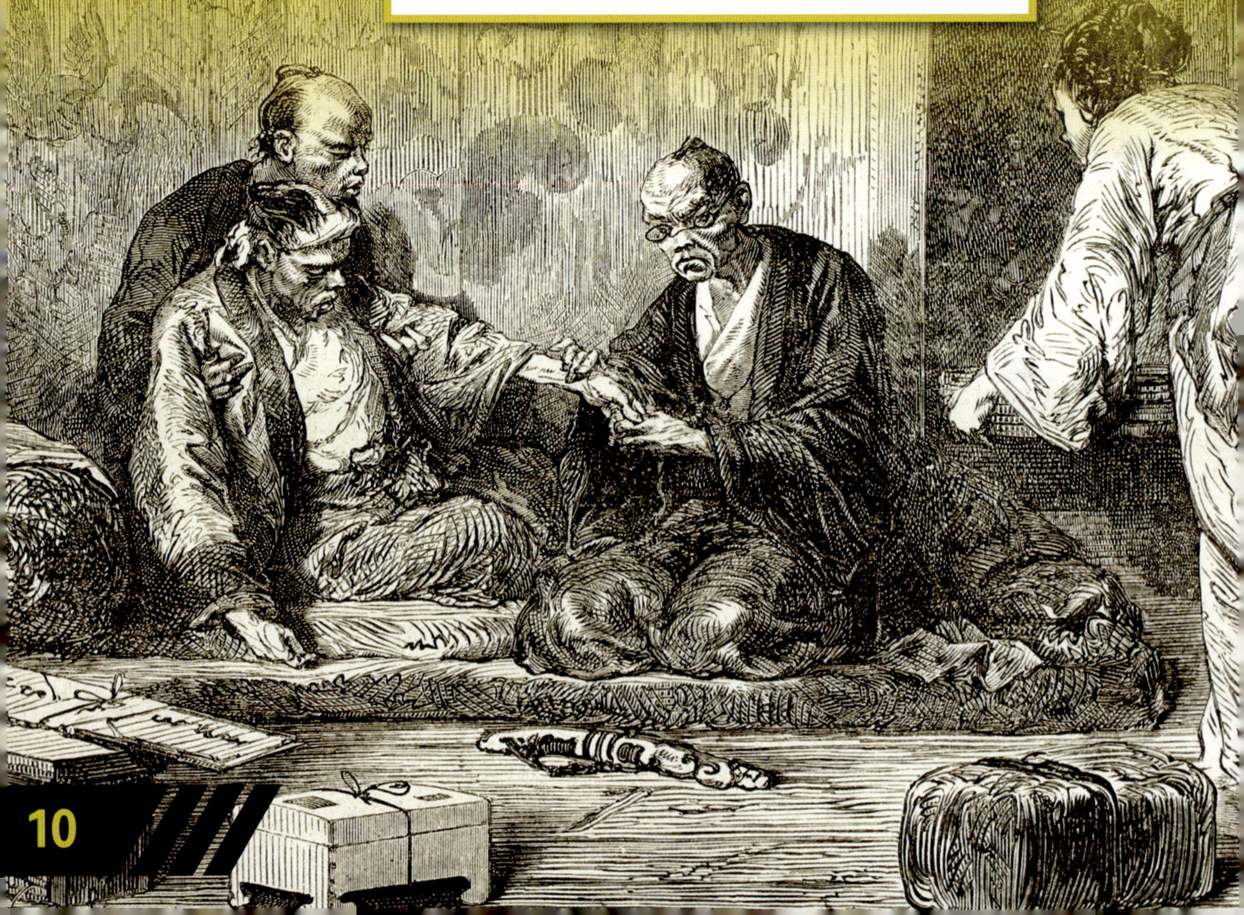

It spreads during wars.

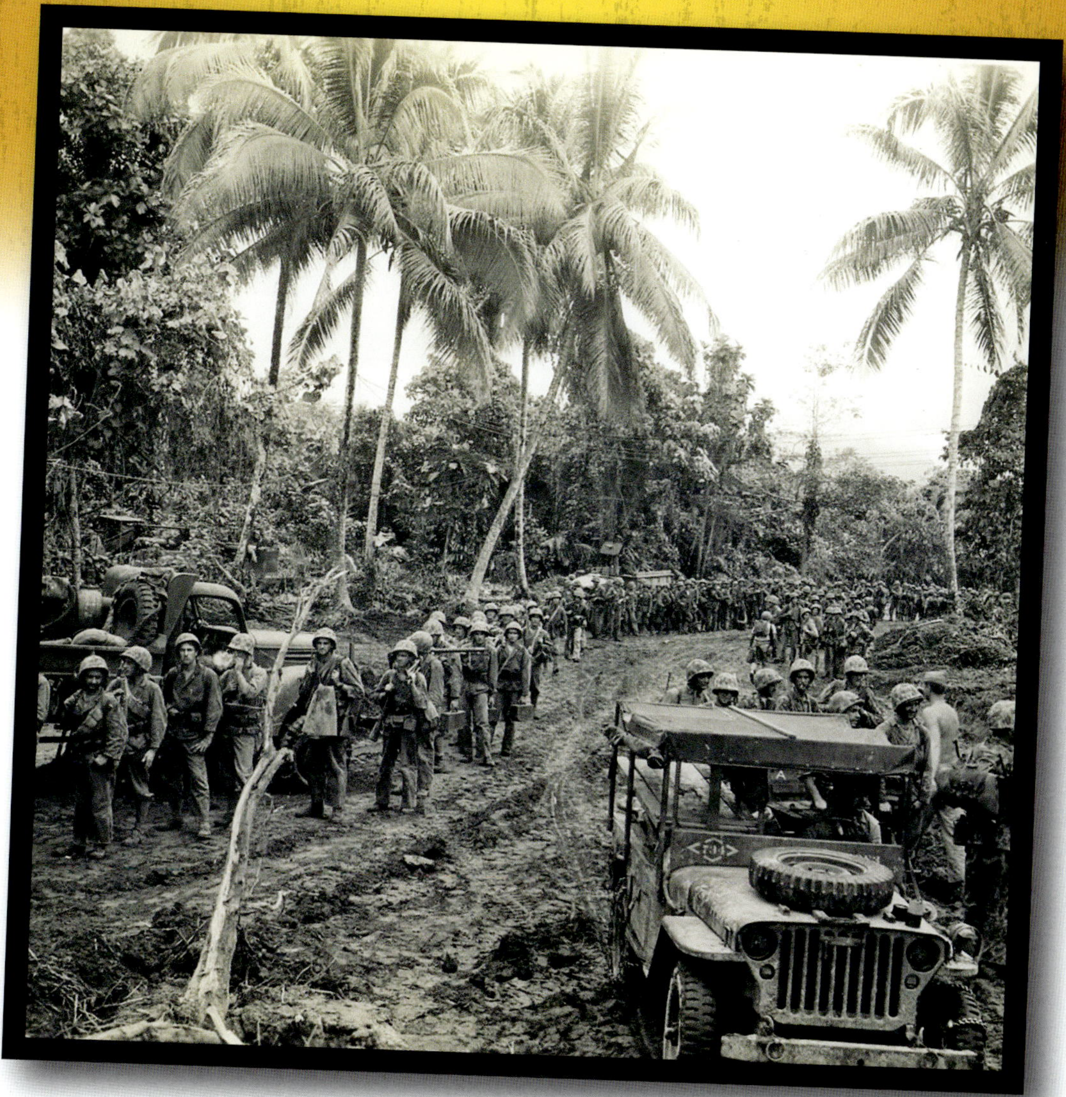

UP CLOSE

The image on the right shows malaria parasites in red blood cells.

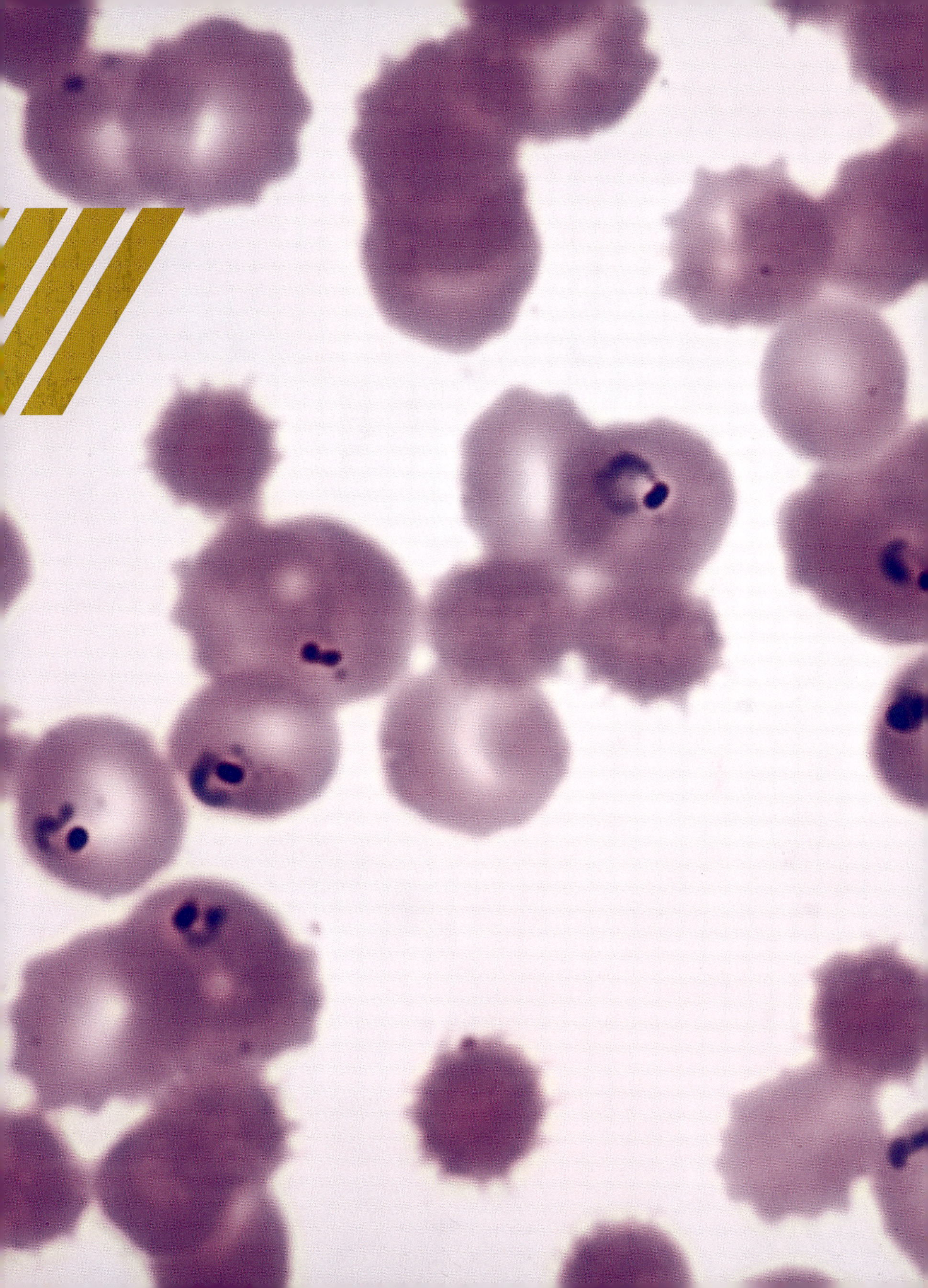

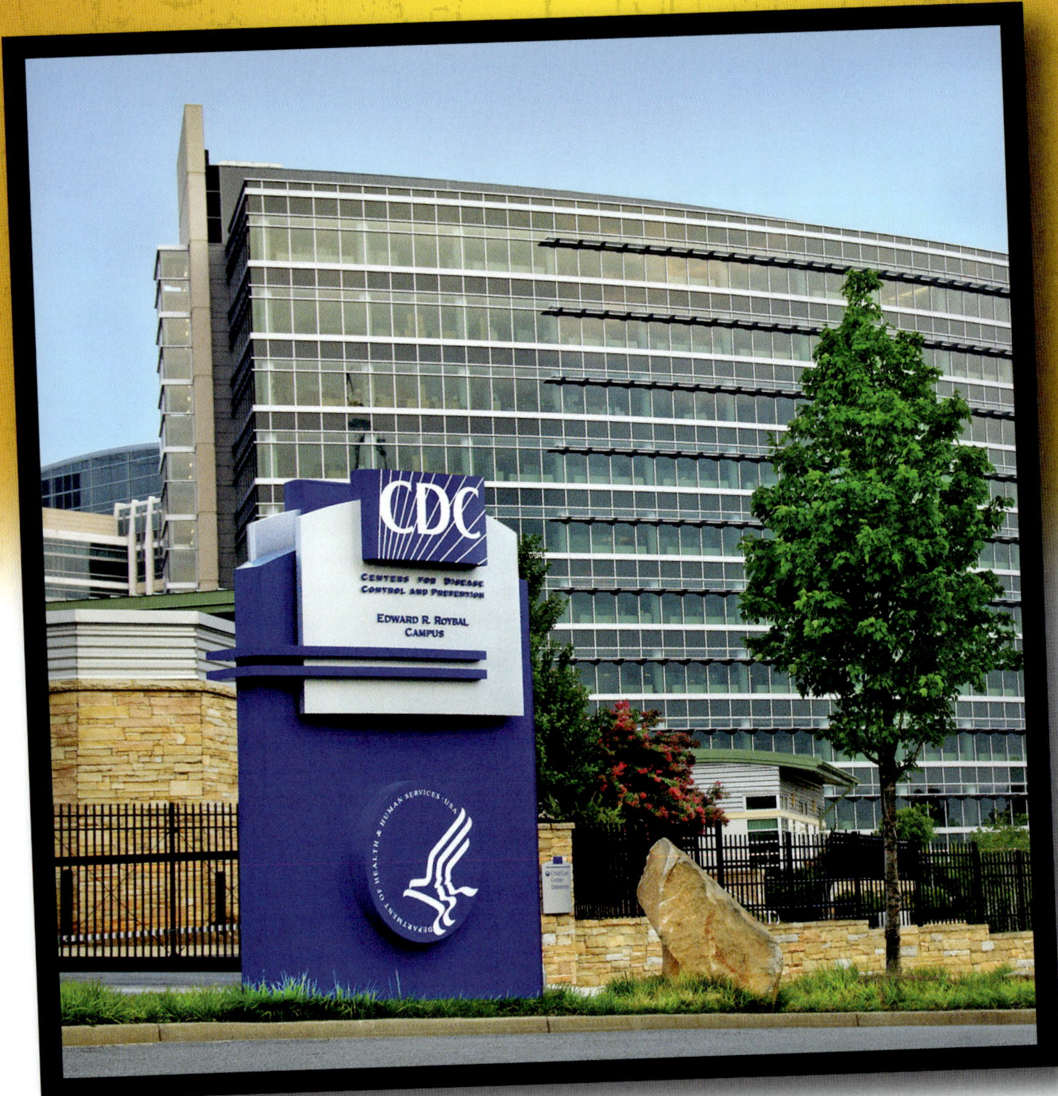

US agencies fight malaria.

agency: a group that provides a service

They look for ways to stop the spread of the disease.

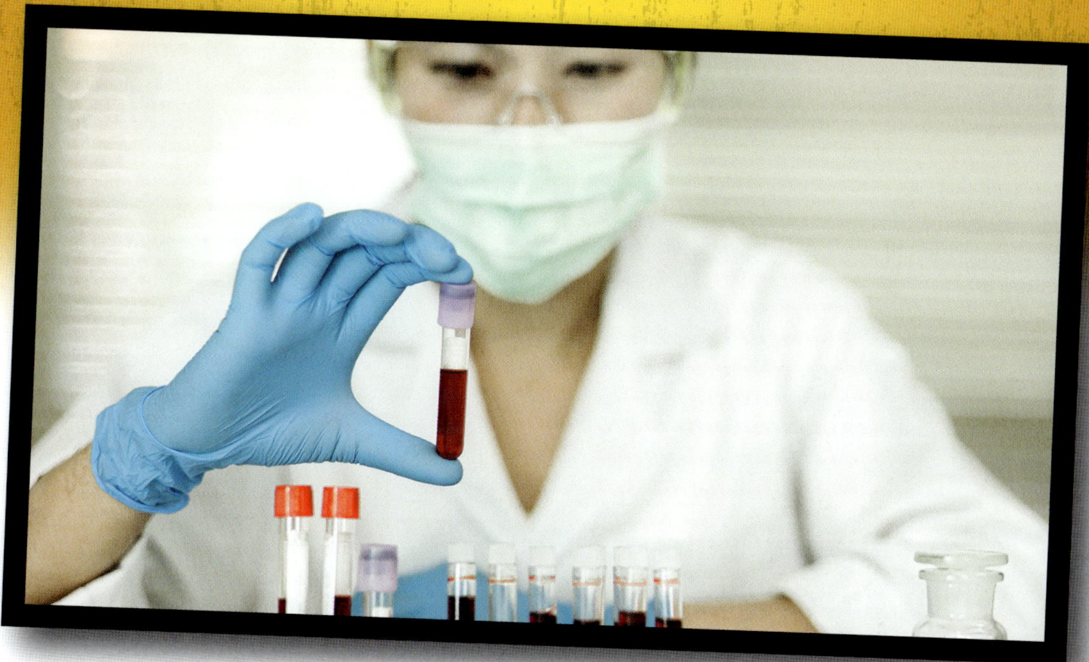

UP NEXT!
Malaria Today.

Malaria Now

We can stay safe from the disease.

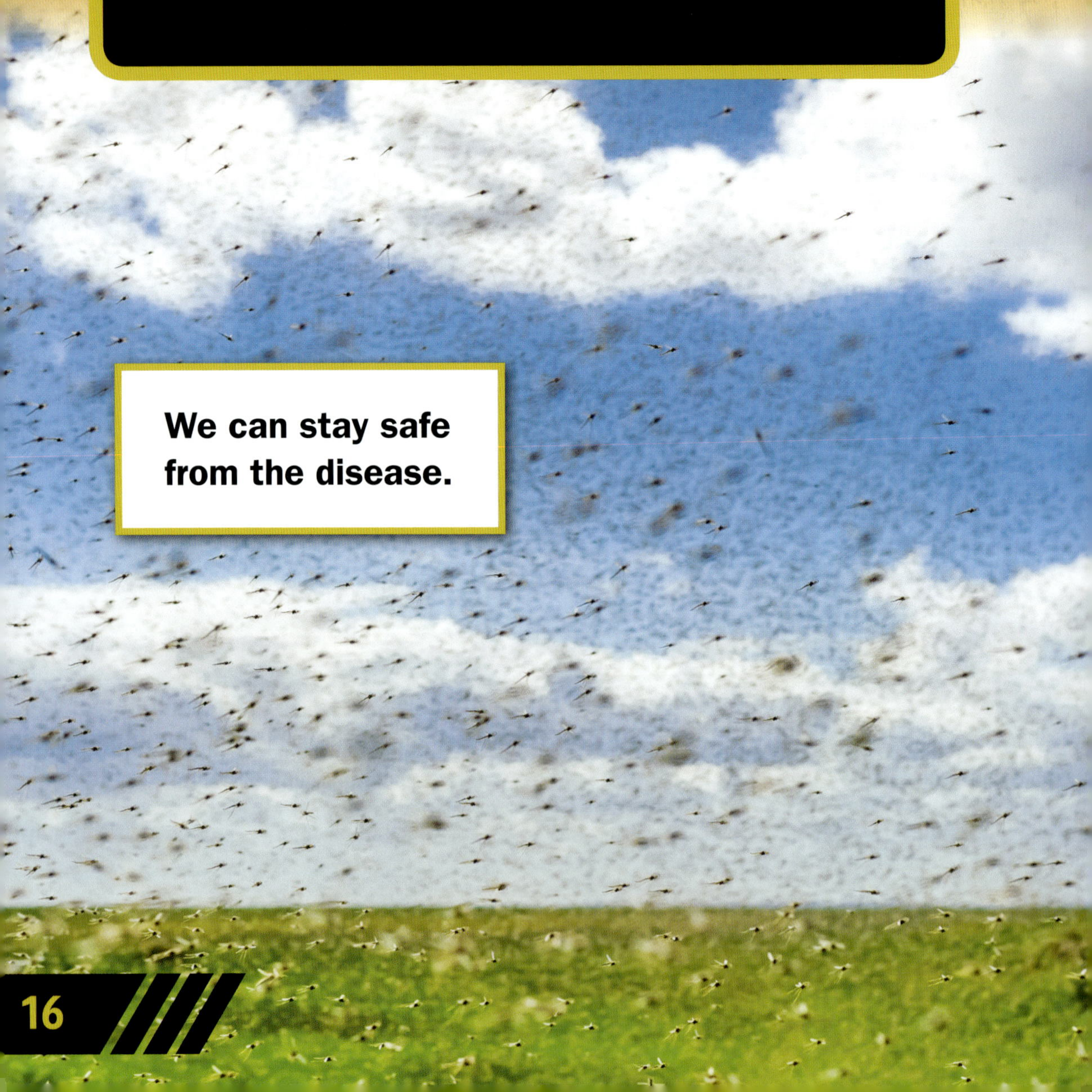

Special nets kill mosquitoes.

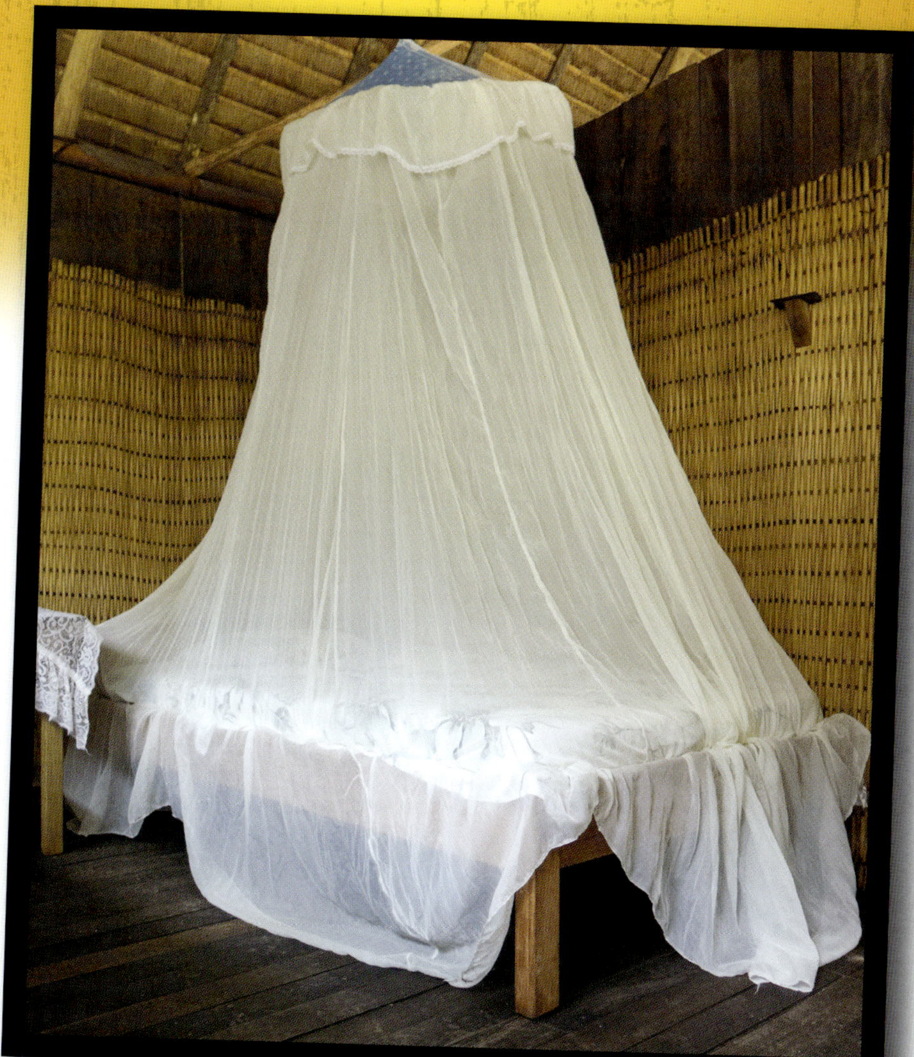

Drugs can treat the disease.

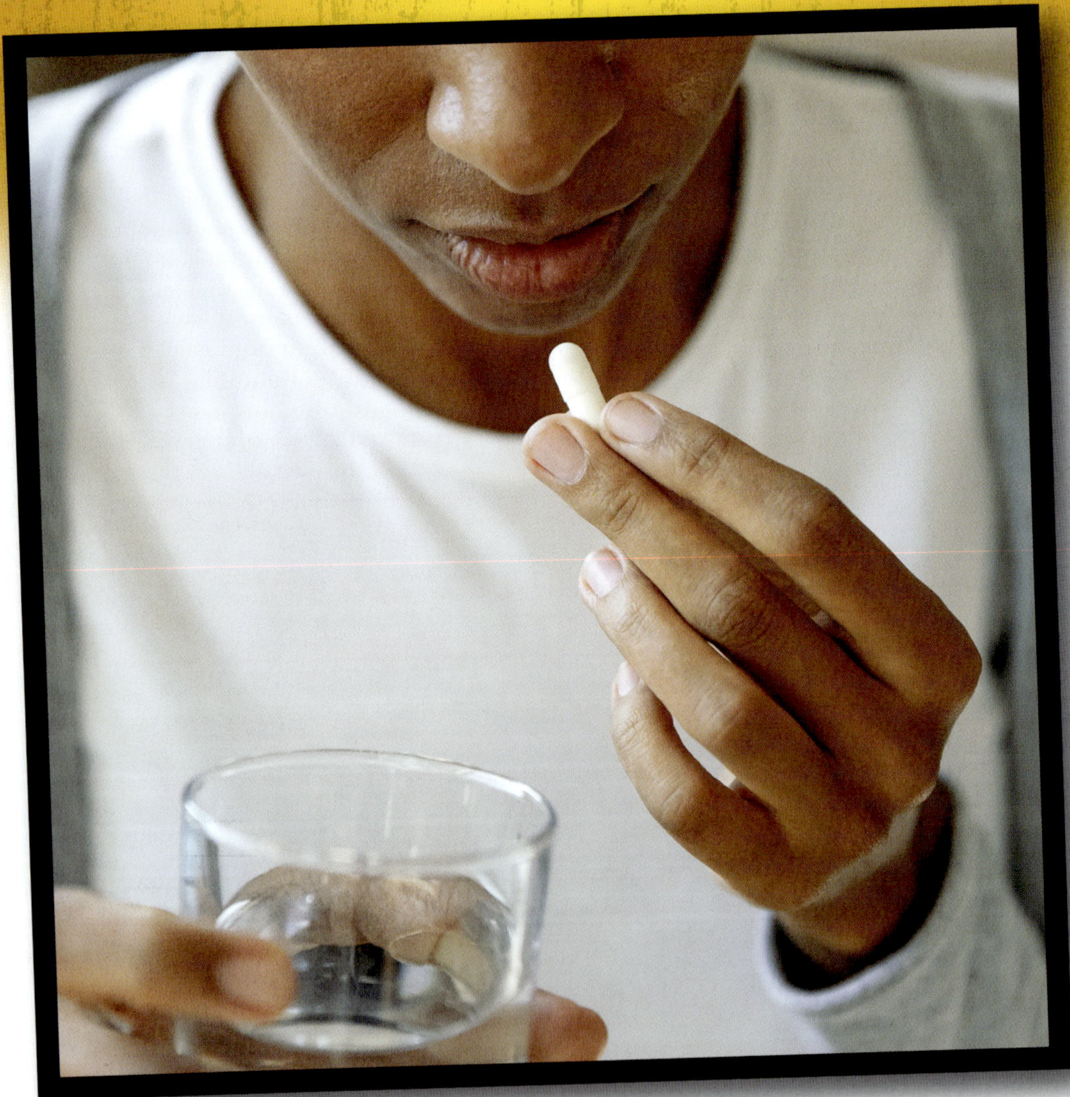

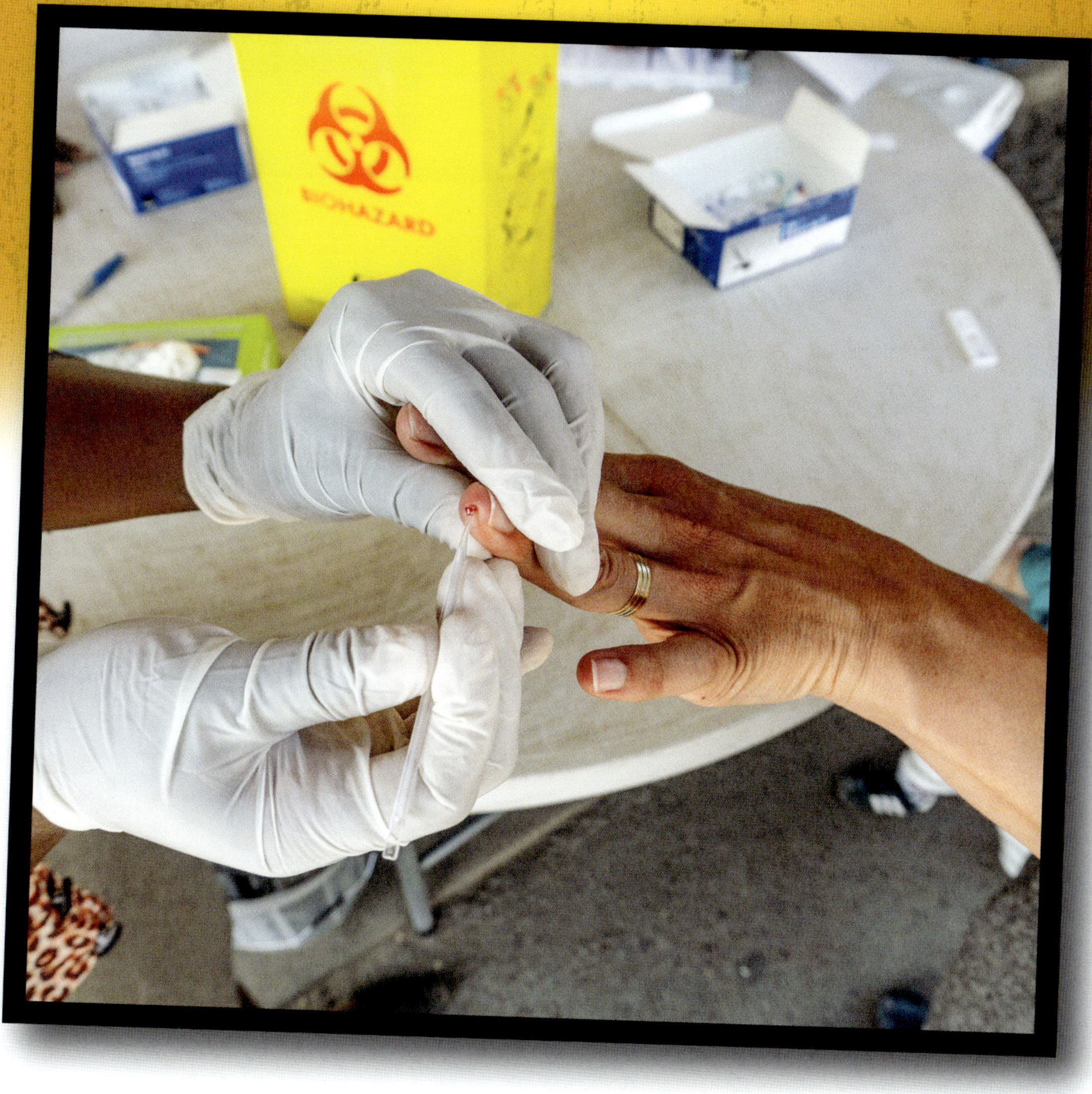

Doctors test people for malaria.

The disease kills fewer people than in the past.

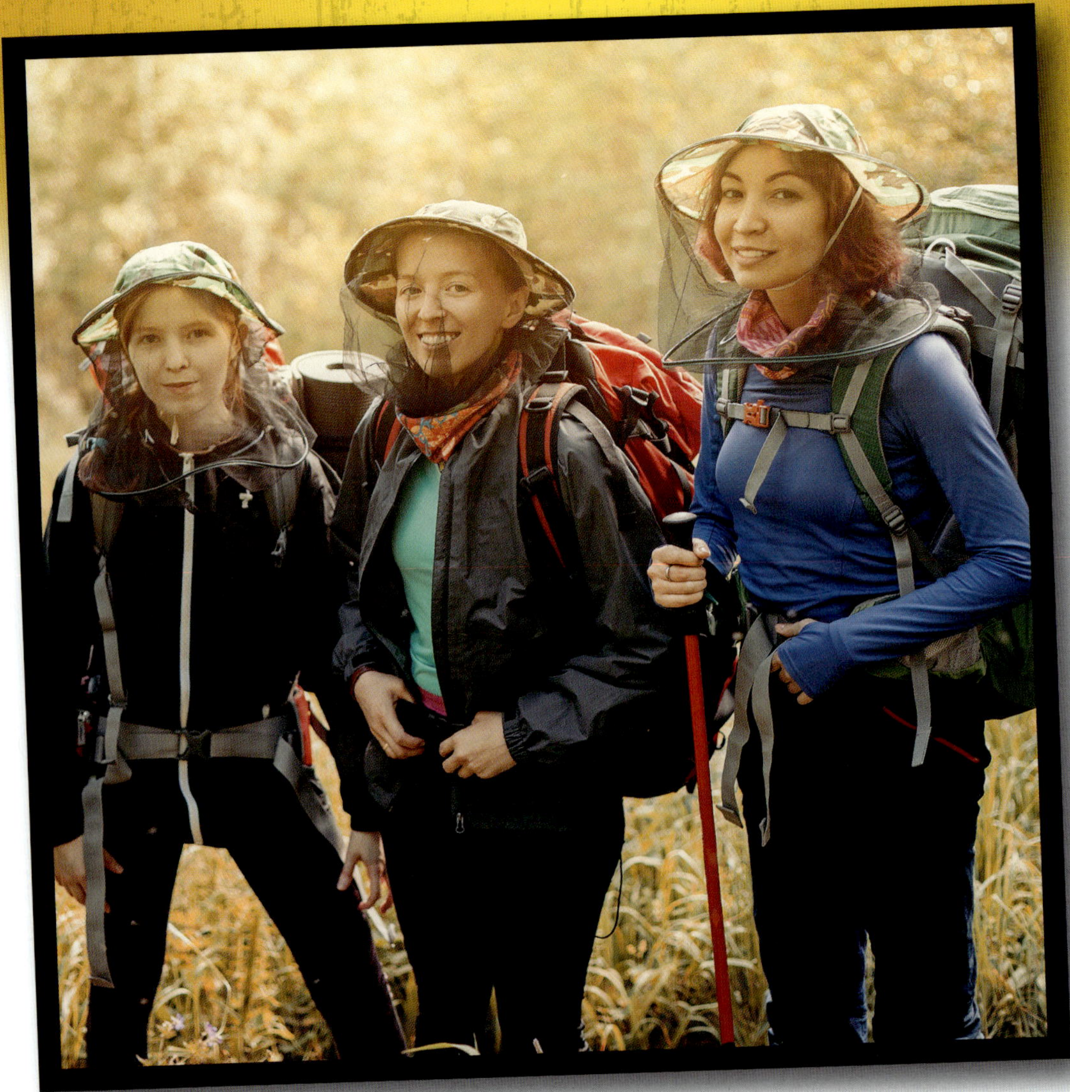

DOCTOR YOU!

Which patient do you think has malaria?

Patient A	Patient B
body ache	cough
fever	fever
headache	headache

Answer: Patient A

Glossary

agency: a group that provides a service

fever: high body temperature

parasite: a living thing that lives on or in another living thing

Check It Out!

Kiddle: Malaria Facts for Kids
https://kids.kiddle.co/Malaria

Leed, Percy. *Bubonic Plague: The Black Death.* Minneapolis: Lerner Publications, 2022.

Markle, Sandra. *Mosquitoes: An Augmented Reality Experience.* Minneapolis: Lerner Publications, 2021.

Mould, Steve. *The Bacteria Book: Gross Germs, Vile Viruses, and Funky Fungi.* New York: DK, 2018.

National Geographic Kids: Mosquito
https://kids.nationalgeographic.com/animals/invertebrates/insects/mosquito/

What Are Germs?
https://kidshealth.org/en/kids/germs.html

Index

Photo Acknowledgments

Image credits: Zadiraka Evgenii/Shutterstock.com, p. 4; Daxiao Productions/Shutterstock.com, p. 5; Maxger/Shutterstock.com, p. 6; xxxstudio/Shutterstock.com, p. 7; GrooveZ/Shutterstock .com, p. 8; namtipStudio/Shutterstock.com, p. 9; Oldtime/Alamy Stock Photo, p. 10; US Marine Corps, p. 11; Ed Reschke/Getty Images, p. 13; Centers for Disease Control and Prevention/ James Gathany, p. 14; Chompoo Suriyo/Shutterstock.com, p. 15; Westend61/Getty Images, p. 16; Toniflap/Shutterstock .com, p. 17; fizkes/Shutterstock.com, p. 18; Sopotnicki/ Shutterstock.com, p. 19; frantic00/Shutterstock.com, p. 20.

Cover: Christoph Burgstedt/Shutterstock.com